CONQUERING
THE GUT

Understanding and Managing

Irritable Bowel Syndrome

Dr. Thomas K. McGlynn

TABLE OF CONTENTS

INTRODUCTION

Irritable Bowel Syndrome, sometimes known simply as IBS, is a prevalent digestive condition that influences the lives of millions of individuals all over the globe. It is a persistent illness that may produce a broad variety of symptoms, some of which include stomach discomfort, bloating, constipation, diarrhea, and changes in bowel habits. Other symptoms include changes in bowel habits. Although irritable bowel syndrome may not cause more severe health issues, it can have a substantial influence on a person's quality of life and ability to function normally during the day.

While the precise causes of irritable bowel syndrome (IBS) are not completely known, research shows that some variables, including genetics, food, stress, and changed gut flora, may all play a part in the condition. Since there are no definitive tests to diagnose IBS, the ailment is often identified via a process known as "elimination." Alterations to one's way of life, medicine, and complementary or alternative treatments are often used in the treatment of irritable bowel syndrome (IBS).

This book seeks to give a thorough reference to understanding irritable bowel syndrome (IBS) and treating its symptoms. In this article, we will talk about the structure and function of the digestive system, the potential causes and triggers of irritable bowel syndrome (IBS), the many forms of IBS, the process of diagnosing IBS, and the numerous treatment options that are available. In addition, we will discuss the impact that food and nutrition have in the management of IBS symptoms, as well as several coping mechanisms that may be used to cope with the illness. This book will provide you with the information and tools you need to effectively manage your symptoms and improve your overall quality of life, regardless of whether you have recently been diagnosed with IBS or have been living with the condition for some time. Its goal is to help you improve your overall quality of life.

In this book, we will discuss the many features of irritable bowel syndrome (IBS) and give guidance and suggestions for effectively treating the illness. Irritable bowel syndrome (IBS) can only be comprehended to a reasonable degree if one has an in-depth knowledge of the structure and operation of the digestive tract, therefore to start, we will go over its architecture and how it operates.

In the next section, we will investigate the variables that might cause or aggravate irritable bowel syndrome (IBS), including anxiety, stress, food, and heredity. If you can identify the specific factors that bring on your IBS symptoms, you will be more equipped to manage them and get them under control.

After that, we will discuss the many subtypes of irritable bowel syndrome (IBS), as well as the diagnostic and therapeutic approaches specific to each subtype. There are three primary subtypes of irritable bowel syndrome (IBS), and it is essential to have a solid understanding of the variations between these subtypes in order to develop the most appropriate treatment strategy.

Alterations to one's way of life, medicine, and complementary or alternative treatments are often used in the treatment of irritable bowel syndrome (IBS). In the following sections, we will examine each of these therapy choices in further depth and provide you with some useful advice for integrating them into your regular practice.

Diet and nutrition are essential components in the management of irritable bowel syndrome (IBS). In this section, we will explore the role that nutrition plays in the management of IBS symptoms and provide advice on foods that should be avoided as well as items that should be included in your diet. In addition, we will go through specific diets for IBS patients, such as the low FODMAP diet, and provide some helpful hints for the planning and preparation of meals.

Last but not least, we will discuss ways for coping with the emotional and psychological effects of irritable bowel syndrome (IBS). IBS is a chronic disease that may be hard to live with; but there are many resources and support groups available to assist you in managing your symptoms and improving your overall quality of life. We hope that by the time you finish reading this book, you will have a better knowledge of irritable bowel syndrome (IBS) and will feel more empowered to take control of your symptoms. Although IBS cannot be cured, it is a disorder that can be managed, and if you have access to the correct resources and assistance, you may have a happy and healthy life despite having this illness.

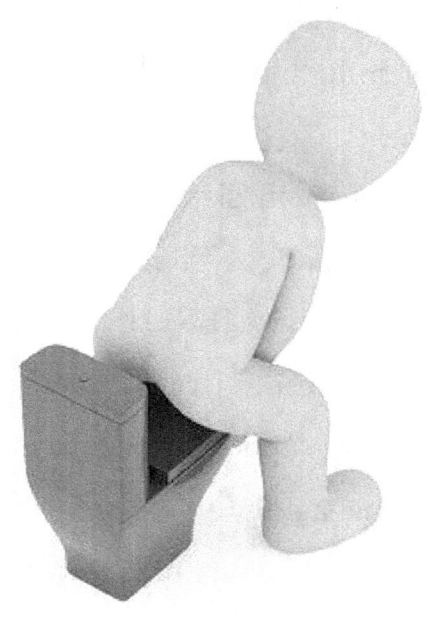

CHAPTER ONE

Irritable Bowel Syndrome (IBS)

Irritable Bowel Syndrome, sometimes known simply as IBS, is a chronic condition of the large intestine that affects the digestive system (colon). It is a functional condition, which means that there are no abnormalities in the digestive system in terms of its physical appearance; nonetheless, the digestive system's function is changed in some manner.

IBS is defined by a variety of symptoms that might differ from one individual to the next but often include stomach discomfort, bloating gas, constipation, diarrhea, or a combination of each of these symptoms. These symptoms may range from moderate to severe, and they have the potential to greatly impair a person's ability to operate normally in day-to-day life.

Research shows that irritable bowel syndrome (IBS) may be caused by a mix of variables, including genetics, changed gut microbiota, nutrition, stress, and anxiety. Nevertheless, the specific etiology of IBS has not been conclusively determined. IBS is a widespread ailment that affects between 10 and 15 percent of the population. While it may strike anyone of any age, young adults are often the ones who are identified as having the condition.

Although IBS does not lead to more significant health issues or damage to the digestive system, it may be a chronic illness that has to be managed on a continuing basis. Alterations to one's way of life, medicine, and complementary and alternative treatments are some of the therapy options that may be used in the management of IBS symptoms. The majority of persons who have irritable bowel syndrome (IBS) are able to successfully control their symptoms and enhance their quality of life with the correct approach.

Irritable bowel syndrome (IBS) is a disorder that may be difficult to treat since it can have a substantial influence on a person's day-to-day life as well as their well-being. Many persons who have irritable bowel syndrome also suffer from emotional and psychological suffering, such as anxiety and depression, in addition to the physical symptoms of the condition.

There are three primary subtypes of irritable bowel syndrome (IBS), and each has a unique collection of symptoms as well as diagnostic criteria. These are the following:

- Constipation, bloating, and stomach discomfort are the hallmarks of irritable bowel syndrome (IBS) with constipation (IBS-C).

- IBS-D, which stands for irritable bowel syndrome with diarrhea, is characterized by diarrhea, urgency, and stomach discomfort.
- Mixed IBS (IBS-M): characterized by a mix of constipation and diarrhea, as well as bloating and stomach discomfort.

Since there are no reliable diagnostic tests for irritable bowel syndrome (IBS), the disorder is often identified via a process of elimination. Inflammatory bowel disease (often known as IBD) and celiac disease are two disorders that might produce symptoms that are very similar to those that you are experiencing. Your doctor may prescribe testing to rule out these other conditions.

Therapy for IBS is customized and may include a mix of lifestyle modifications, medicines, and other treatments. Modifications to one's nutrition, methods of stress reduction, and consistent physical activity are all examples of possible lifestyle adjustments. Laxatives, antispasmodics, and antidepressants are all potential treatment options for irritable bowel syndrome (IBS). It's possible that alternative treatments like acupuncture and probiotics might assist some individuals with irritable bowel syndrome (IBS).

The symptoms of irritable bowel syndrome (IBS) may be effectively managed by the use of a variety of medicinal therapies as well as several self-help options. They may include maintaining a symptom journal, identifying and avoiding trigger foods, practicing relaxation methods, and getting help from a healthcare professional or support group.

In general, irritable bowel syndrome (IBS) is a disease that may be difficult to live with; however, with the appropriate strategy and support, the vast majority of individuals who have IBS can successfully manage their symptoms and improve their quality of life.

The Prevalence Of IBS

Irritable bowel syndrome (also known as IBS) is a prevalent gastrointestinal condition that affects between 10 and 15 percent of the population globally. It often starts in the early stages of adulthood and is far more prevalent in females than in males.

Irritable bowel syndrome (IBS) is one of the most prevalent gastrointestinal illnesses and is believed to affect somewhere between 25 and 45 million individuals in the United States. It is also one of the most common reasons why individuals seek medical treatment for digestive issues.

Irritable bowel syndrome (IBS) is a disorder that does not pose a danger to a person's life, but it may have a substantial negative effect on a person's quality of life by causing a person to experience physical pain, social shame, and mental misery. Irritable bowel syndrome (IBS) may cause symptoms that are persistent and unexpected, which can result in lost time at work or school and reduced overall productivity.

Many people with irritable bowel syndrome (IBS), despite its prevalence, do not seek medical care or receive a diagnosis, either because they are ashamed to talk about their symptoms or because they are unaware that their symptoms are related to a medical condition. One of the reasons for this could be that they are unaware that their symptoms are related to a medical condition. This underscores how important it is to educate people about irritable bowel syndrome (IBS) as well as the availability of medicines that are beneficial in controlling the illness.

There are a number of variables that might put a person at a higher risk of having irritable bowel syndrome (IBS). These are the following:

Age: Irritable bowel syndrome is often diagnosed in young adults; however, the condition may strike anyone of any age.

Gender: Women have a higher risk of developing irritable bowel syndrome than men do.

Family history: irritable bowel syndrome (IBS) is more likely to develop in those who have a family history of the condition or other gastrointestinal problems.

Psychological factors: irritable bowel syndrome (IBS) has been related to psychological issues such as stress, anxiety, and depression.

Gut microbiota: irritable bowel syndrome (IBS) may be caused, at least in part, by an imbalance in the microbiota that lives in the gut, according to research.

Food sensitivities and intolerances: Some persons who have irritable bowel syndrome (IBS) may have food sensitivities or intolerances that cause their symptoms.

Research shows that irritable bowel syndrome (IBS) may be associated with abnormal communication between the brain and the stomach, however, the specific etiology of the condition is not completely known. This connection is sometimes referred to as the gut-brain axis, and it includes intricate interactions between the enteric nervous system, the central nervous system, and the gut microbiota. The enteric neural system is responsible for controlling the digestive system.

Research has also indicated that persons who have irritable bowel syndrome may have a higher sensitivity to particular stimuli in the digestive tract, such as gas or stool, which may cause symptoms to become activated. It is believed that alterations in the way the nervous system processes and reacts to these stimuli are to blame for this hypersensitivity.

Irritable bowel syndrome is thought to be a complicated condition that is brought on by a number of different variables, despite the fact that its precise origins are still a mystery and cannot be completely explained. Managing symptoms and increasing quality of life are the primary goals of treatment for irritable bowel syndrome (IBS). This treatment may entail making adjustments to one's lifestyle, taking medication, or participating in alternative treatments.

Common Symptoms of IBS

Irritable bowel syndrome (IBS) is characterized by a variety of symptoms, some of which include the following:

Pain or discomfort in the abdomen: This condition is often characterized as a cramping or a sharp ache in the lower abdomen. It's possible that passing stool or gas can help reduce the discomfort.

Bloating: The term "bloating" refers to a sensation of fullness or tightness in the abdominal region, which may be accompanied by apparent swelling or distention of the abdominal region.

Alterations in bowel habits: They may take the form of either diarrhea or constipation, or they can be a mix of the two. Individuals who have IBS are more likely to have bowel motions that are either urgent or incomplete.

Gas: Because of this, you may have belly pain or bloating. Gas.

Mucus in the stool: The presence of mucus in the stool is an indication that there may be inflammation in the digestive system.

Nausea: Nausea may be described as a queasy sensation or an overwhelming need to throw up.

Fatigue: Fatigue is a common symptom of irritable bowel syndrome (IBS), which may be caused by irregular sleep habits or the stress caused by living with IBS.

Anxiety or depression: Anxiety and depression are two of the most prevalent psychological symptoms of irritable bowel syndrome (IBS). These conditions may be linked to the stress and disturbance that are generated by the ailment.

It is essential to keep in mind that the intensity of the symptoms and the frequency with which they occur might vary greatly from one individual to the next. Some individuals may have moderate symptoms that may not substantially impair their day-to-day living, while others may have more severe symptoms that need medical care as well as alterations to their way of life. If you are having any of these symptoms, you should make an appointment with your primary care physician as soon as possible in order to rule out any other possible causes and to build a treatment strategy for managing your symptoms.

Irritable bowel syndrome is characterized by relapsing and remitting symptoms throughout time, with periods of remission (in which symptoms are less severe or nonexistent) alternating with times of flare-ups. This is one of the defining characteristics of IBS (when symptoms are more severe). Symptoms may be brought on or made worse by a variety of reasons, including the following:

Diet: Some individuals are more likely to have symptoms of irritable bowel syndrome (IBS) if they consume dairy products, high-fat meals, coffee, or alcohol.

Stress: Some persons who have IBS are more susceptible to having their symptoms triggered or made worse by emotional or psychological stress.

Hormonal changes: irritable bowel syndrome (IBS) symptoms might fluctuate depending on a woman's menstrual cycle because of hormonal shifts.

Medications: Some drugs, such as antibiotics, have been shown to upset the natural balance of bacteria in the stomach, which may result in IBS symptoms.

Infections: In some patients, symptoms of IBS may be triggered by infections in the gastrointestinal tract.

It is also essential to remember that some individuals who have IBS may suffer symptoms that are not connected to the digestive system, such as headaches, back pain, or urine problems. This is something that should be taken into consideration. These symptoms are referred to as "extra-intestinal" or "non-gastrointestinal" symptoms, and they may be connected to the effect that IBS has on the neurological system or other bodily systems.

In general, irritable bowel syndrome (IBS) is a complicated and diverse disorder that may have a considerable influence on the quality of life of a person. Yet, many individuals who have IBS are able to control their symptoms and lead productive lives after receiving an accurate diagnosis and treatment for their condition.

The Influence that IBS has on One's Quality of Life

Research has shown that irritable bowel syndrome (IBS) may have a substantial influence on a person's social and personal life. This might cause the individual to avoid particular settings or activities out of fear of experiencing symptoms or feeling embarrassed. Because of this, a person's quality of life may suffer, and they may become socially isolated. A person who suffers from irritable bowel syndrome (IBS) may, for instance, try to avoid situations in which their symptoms are likely to become worse, such as going out to dine with friends or family, traveling, or engaging in strenuous activities.

In addition, persons who have IBS symptoms more often or severely may have a worse quality of life as a result of the condition. According to a number of studies, those who suffer from more severe cases of

IBS have a worse quality of life and higher levels of mental distress compared to those whose symptoms are less severe. Individuals who have IBS and also have other medical diseases or psychological disorders, such as anxiety or depression, may also be at a higher risk of having their quality of life deteriorate.

IBS may have a substantial impact on quality of life; however, there are numerous treatment options available to help control symptoms and improve overall well-being. It is crucial to highlight that despite this fact, IBS can be effectively managed and treated. Alterations to one's diet, methods of stress management, prescribed medicine, and talk therapy are all potential options. Those who suffer from irritable bowel syndrome (IBS) should work closely with their healthcare physician to devise a tailored treatment plan that takes into account their unique symptoms and requirements.

IBS may have a substantial effect, both physically and emotionally, on a person's quality of life. Irritable bowel syndrome (IBS) is a digestive disorder that may cause its sufferers to experience a variety of symptoms that vary from severe to unpleasant to life-disrupting. These symptoms may also be humiliating, which can lead to feelings of worry as well as social isolation.

IBS may have an effect not only on a person's physical symptoms but also on their mental well-being. The inability to accurately foresee one's symptoms, along with the need of making plans around those symptoms, maybe a source of stress, which in turn can lead to anxiety, sadness, or other psychological problems. Individuals who have irritable bowel syndrome may also have trouble sleeping or keeping up with their normal exercise routines, all of which may have a negative influence on their overall quality of life.

The influence of irritable bowel syndrome on one's quality of life might extend to one's professional or academic life. Individuals who have IBS may find that their symptoms require them to miss time at work or school, or they may find that they are less productive or have a harder time focusing owing to the discomfort or pain they are experiencing.

The influence that irritable bowel syndrome has on a person's quality of life may be somewhat variable as a whole, depending on the intensity of the symptoms, the person's capacity to control them, and the existence of other medical or psychiatric illnesses. It is essential for persons who have irritable bowel syndrome (IBS) to seek help from healthcare experts, members of their families, or support groups in order to better manage their symptoms and enhance their overall well-being.

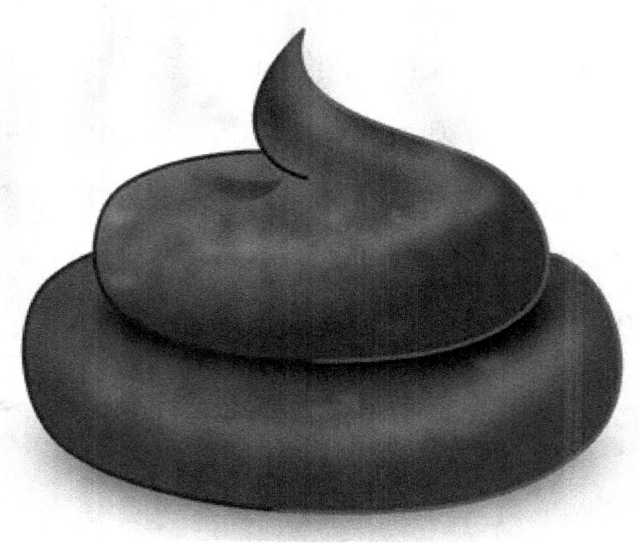

CHAPTER TWO

Understanding the Digestive System

It is essential to have a fundamental knowledge of the digestive system in order to comprehend irritable bowel syndrome (IBS). It is the job of the digestive system to convert the nutrients in food into a form that can be absorbed by the body and put to use there. It is composed of a number of organs and structures, such as the mouth, the esophagus, the stomach, the small intestine, the large intestine (sometimes called the colon), the rectum, and the anus.

After being swallowed, food makes its way down the esophagus and into the stomach, where it is combined with digestive enzymes and acids. This is the beginning of the digestive process. After that, it travels to the small intestine, which is part of the digestive tract where the vast majority of the nutrients are absorbed into circulation. The leftover waste materials are subsequently removed via the rectum and the anus after passing through the large intestine. Here, they are transformed into feces before being expelled from the body.

The digestive tract is also home to a diverse community of bacteria known as the gut microbiome. These microbes are known to play a vital role in digestion, the absorption of nutrients, and the operation of the immune system. A person's food, the drugs they take, and the way they live their lives all have an impact on the microbiome that lives in their gut. This microbiome is made up of trillions of bacteria, viruses, fungi, and other types of microorganisms.

In persons who suffer from irritable bowel syndrome (IBS), the microbiome of the gut may be disrupted or out of balance, which may be a factor in the development of symptoms such as abdominal discomfort, bloating, and irregular bowel movements. In order to develop successful treatment techniques for irritable bowel syndrome (IBS), it is necessary to make significant progress in understanding the role that the digestive system and the gut flora play in the disorder.

The Structure and Function of the Digestive System
It is important to keep in mind that the digestive system is a very intricate and linked system and that there are a variety of things that may affect the way in which it works. For instance, the nervous system is responsible for a significant portion of the work involved in the regulation of digestion. Specifically, signals sent from the brain and spinal cord contribute to the management of how food is moved through the digestive tract. In addition, the endocrine system contributes, with hormones like gastrin and cholecystokinin helping to control the

number of digestive enzymes and acids that are produced in the body.

In addition, digestion and general health are both affected by the gut microbiome, which is comprised of billions of bacteria that reside in the digestive system and play a vital role in maintaining its balance. The microbiome in the gut not only serves to control the immune system and guard against pathogenic bacteria and viruses, but it also plays a role in the digestion of food and the extraction of nutrients.

Those who have IBS may have problems or imbalances in any of these systems, which may result in symptoms such as stomach discomfort, bloating, and irregular bowel patterns. Irritable bowel syndrome (IBS) is a common digestive disorder that may be difficult to diagnose and treat effectively without first having a thorough grasp of the many variables that contribute to it.

The digestive system is a complicated system that is composed of several organs and structures, each of which performs a specific job that is essential to the body. The following is a concise summary of the anatomy pertaining to the digestive system:

Mouth: The first step in digestion takes place in the mouth. When chewing, saliva, which includes enzymes that begin the process of breaking down carbs, is combined with the food being chewed.

The esophagus: is a muscular tube that runs from the mouth down to the stomach. It links the two cavities. Contraction of the muscles helps move food into the stomach after it has been swallowed.

The stomach: is a muscular sac that combines and grinds food with digesting enzymes and acids. The stomach is located in the middle of the digestive tract. This assists in the process of converting food into chyme, which has a liquid consistency.

Small intestine: The small intestine is a lengthy tube that runs from the stomach all the way down to the big intestine. It connects the two. It is via this process that the majority of the nutrients that are taken in through food are absorbed into the bloodstream. The duodenum, the jejunum, and the ileum make up the small intestine, which is separated into three portions.

Large intestine (colon): The large intestine is a tube that is bigger than the small intestine and is responsible for generating solid stools by absorbing water and electrolytes from the residual chyme. The rectum is responsible for the storage of feces before they are expelled via the anus.

The liver is responsible for the production of bile, which is then stored in the gallbladder. Bile plays an important role in the digestion of lipids in the small intestine.

The pancreas: is responsible for the production of digestive enzymes, which are then secreted into the small intestine where they assist in the further digestion of food.

The appendix: is a tiny finger-like extensor from the big intestine that is known as the appendix. Its purpose is not entirely clear; however, it is thought to be involved with the body's immune system in some way.

Irritable bowel syndrome (IBS) is one of the digestive conditions that may be helped by having a better understanding of the architecture of the digestive system, which can assist locate the issue and rule out probable causes.

The Functioning of the Digestive System

It is the job of the digestive system to convert the nutrients in food into a form that can be absorbed by the body and put to use there. The following is a concise explanation of how the digestive system functions:

Ingestion: Chewing the food first brings it into the mouth, where it is then swallowed after being broken up into tiny pieces.

Digestion: The process of digestion begins when food moves from the mouth through the lower esophagus and then into the stomach. Once there, the food is combined with digestive enzymes and acids. This contributes to the process of breaking down the meal into smaller molecules that the body is able to absorb.

Absorption: The small intestine is responsible for the majority of the body's ability to absorb nutrients. Villi are finger-like projections that are found on the inner surface of the walls of the small intestine. These villi help to expand the surface area of the small intestine, which in turn facilitates the absorption of nutrients into the bloodstream.

Elimination: The leftover waste materials are transported to the large intestine, where they stay until they are combined with water and electrolytes to form solid feces. The rectum is responsible for the storage of feces before they are expelled via the anus.

A complicated interaction of hormones, enzymes, and nerve impulses is responsible for the regulation of the digestive and absorption processes. For instance, when there is food in the stomach, the hormone gastrin is secreted, which increases the synthesis of stomach acid and digesting enzymes. Another example is when there is food in the stomach, the hormone leptin is secreted. The mouth is where the enzyme amylase is secreted, which begins the process of breaking down carbohydrates. The small intestine is where the enzymes lipase and protease are secreted, which break down fats and proteins respectively.

A healthy gut microbiome is essential to the proper functioning of the digestive system. The gut microbiome is made up of billions of bacteria that reside in the digestive tract. The microbiome in the gut not only serves to control the immune system and guard against pathogenic bacteria and viruses, but it also plays a role in the digestion of food and the extraction of nutrients.

Symptoms of irritable bowel syndrome (IBS) might include stomach discomfort, bloating, and irregular bowel movements. These symptoms can be caused by disruptions or imbalances in the digestive tract or the gut flora, respectively. In order to create successful treatment techniques for irritable bowel syndrome (IBS), it is necessary to first have a solid understanding of how the digestive system functions.

The Importance of the Microbiota in the Gut

The digestive tract is home to a diverse community of bacteria that make up what is known as the gut microbiome. It is expected to include trillions upon trillions of cells, and its constituents include bacteria, viruses, fungi, and other microbes.

The microbiome of the gut plays a crucial part in digestion, as it contributes to the process of breaking down food and obtaining the nutrients that the body requires. In addition to this, it is very important for the regulation of the immune system and the defense against hazardous infections.

In addition, research has revealed that the microbiome of the gut may have an effect on a broad spectrum of health outcomes, ranging from metabolic problems and obesity to mental health conditions and neurological illnesses.

IBS is a condition that affects the gut microbiota and may cause indications such as stomach discomfort, bloating, and irregular bowel movements. These symptoms can be caused by disruptions or imbalances in the gut microbiome. For instance, some research has shown that persons who suffer from irritable bowel syndrome may have fewer quantities of certain helpful bacteria in the stomach, while other research has suggested that they may have larger numbers of dangerous bacteria.

It is not yet known how alterations to the gut microbiota may be utilized to treat or prevent irritable bowel syndrome (IBS), since researchers are currently investigating the intricate relationship that exists between the gut microbiome and IBS. On the other hand, there is a rising interest in the possibility of probiotics and other therapies to regulate the gut microbiota and alleviate symptoms in persons who have irritable bowel syndrome (IBS).

The examination of the microbiome of the intestines and its possible function in irritable bowel syndrome (IBS) is still in its infancy, but there are several intriguing avenues of inquiry to pursue. For instance, a number of studies have shown that certain probiotics could be useful in alleviating the symptoms of irritable bowel syndrome (IBS).

Probiotics are living microorganisms that are analogous to the helpful bacteria that are already present in the human digestive tract and are found naturally. You may get them in the form of supplements, or you can find them naturally occurring in foods like yogurt and kefir.

Some strains of probiotics, such as Bifidobacterium infantis and Lactobacillus plantarum, were shown to be useful in lowering the symptoms of irritable bowel syndrome (IBS), according to a study that analyzed the results of 19 randomized controlled trials. Nevertheless, the precise probiotic strains and doses that are most beneficial for treating irritable bowel syndrome might differ from one individual to the next.

Other interventions, such as fecal microbiota transplantation (FMT), which involves transplanting fecal matter from a healthy donor into the gut of a person who has a dysbiotic gut microbiome, may also help to modulate the gut microbiome and improve the symptoms of irritable bowel syndrome (IBS). Prebiotics are a type of fiber that helps to feed the beneficial bacteria that are already present in the gut.

Although research on these therapies is still ongoing and they are not currently commonly utilized to treat IBS, the possibilities they provide for future research and treatment choices are quite encouraging. Improved knowledge of the gut microbiota and the role it plays in irritable bowel syndrome (IBS) might, in the long run, lead to more effective and individualized therapies for this complicated ailment.

CHAPTER THREE

Causes and Triggers of IBS

Research has uncovered a number of probable variables that may contribute to the development of irritable bowel syndrome (IBS); however, the specific etiology of the ailment is not completely known. These are the following:

Problems with the axis between the stomach and the brain: A sophisticated network of nerves, hormones, and other signaling molecules establishes a connection between the digestive tract and the brain. Several researchers are of the opinion that irritable bowel syndrome (IBS) may be caused, at least in part, by an imbalance in the gut-brain axis.

Inflammation in the intestines: Some research has shown that the presence of chronic low-grade inflammation in the intestines may contribute to the development of irritable bowel syndrome (IBS).

Irregularities or disruptions in the gut microbiome: As was discussed previously, irregularities or disturbances in the gut microbiota may be a factor in the development of IBS symptoms.

Food sensitivities and intolerances: Some people who have irritable bowel syndrome (IBS) may have a sensitivity or intolerance to particular kinds of foods, such as dairy products, gluten, or FODMAPs (fermentable oligo-, di-, and monosaccharides and polyols), which are different kinds of carbohydrates that are poorly absorbed in the small intestine.

Tension and nervousness: While stress and worry are not thought to be the primary cause of irritable bowel syndrome (IBS), studies have shown that they may make the symptoms of the illness worse for some individuals who have it.

In addition to these possible contributing variables, there are also a number of triggers that, when present, may cause symptoms of irritable bowel syndrome (IBS) to become more severe. They may include the following:

Certain foods: As was discussed before, it is possible that some persons who have IBS are hypersensitive or intolerant to certain kinds of foods.

Hormonal changes: Symptom shifts may occur throughout a woman's menstrual cycle if she has irritable bowel syndrome due to hormonal fluctuations.

Anxiety and stress: The symptoms of irritable bowel syndrome (IBS) may be made worse by worry and stress, as was noted before.

Medication: Patients who have irritable bowel syndrome (IBS) may have a worsening of their symptoms after taking certain medicines, including antibiotics and nonsteroidal anti-inflammatory drugs (NSAIDs).

Alterations in routine: Alterations in routine, such as going on vacation or beginning a new job, might make symptoms worse for some individuals who have irritable bowel syndrome (IBS).

Irritable bowel syndrome (IBS) risk factors

There are a number of variables that have been recognized as having the potential to have a role in the development of irritable bowel syndrome, including the following:

Genetics: There is some evidence from studies that show that irritable bowel syndrome (IBS) may have a hereditary component; however, the specific genes implicated are not yet completely known.

Abnormalities in the movement of the gut: Changes in bowel habits and symptoms may occur in certain persons who have irritable bowel syndrome (IBS) because the muscles in the gut might contract abnormally vigorously or weakly in these patients.

Changes in gut bacteria: Alterations in the bacteria of the gut as was indicated previously, irritable bowel syndrome (IBS) may be caused in part by disruptions or imbalances in the microbiome of the gut.

Inflammation in the intestines: Some research has shown that the presence of chronic low-grade inflammation in the intestines may contribute to the development of irritable bowel syndrome (IBS).

Visceral hypersensitivity: irritable bowel syndrome (IBS) is a group of symptoms that may be brought on by a condition known as visceral hypersensitivity, which describes a heightened sensitivity to pain and discomfort in the gastrointestinal tract.

Stress and anxiety: While stress and worry are not thought to be a direct cause of irritable bowel syndrome (IBS), studies have shown that they may make the symptoms of the illness worse for some individuals who already have it.

Trauma or abuse: Those who have been physically, emotionally, or sexually abused or who have been the victims of traumatic events are more prone to acquire irritable bowel syndrome, according to the findings of some research.

Changes in hormone levels: As was noted previously, women who suffer from irritable bowel syndrome may notice a shift in their symptoms throughout their menstrual cycle.

Infections: In some individuals, the beginning symptoms of irritable bowel syndrome (IBS) may be triggered by certain bacterial or viral illnesses of the stomach, such as gastroenteritis.

It is essential to keep in mind that not all persons who have irritable bowel syndrome (IBS) have the same contributing variables, and in many instances, the precise etiology of the ailment is not entirely known. People who have irritable bowel syndrome (IBS) may improve their symptoms and their quality of life overall by identifying and treating the probable variables that contribute to their condition.

Frequent causes of symptoms of irritable bowel syndrome

IBS symptoms may be triggered by a wide variety of factors, however, there are a few frequent triggers that are mentioned by many individuals who have IBS. These are the following:

Several foods, including irritable bowel syndrome (IBS) symptoms, may be brought on in some individuals by certain kinds of meals. Dairy products, meals containing gluten, foods rich in fat, foods strong in spice, caffeine, alcohol, and artificial sweeteners are common allergens that may set off an allergic reaction.

Anxiety and stress: Anxiety and stress may be a cause for IBS symptoms, or they can make existing symptoms worse. It's possible that this is related to the fact that stress and worry may have an effect on the motility of the intestines, as well as inflammation and visceral sensitivity.

Changes in hormone levels: It is possible for women who suffer from irritable bowel syndrome to notice a shift in their symptoms throughout their menstrual cycle. This shift may be due to hormonal shifts.

Medications: Antibiotics and other nonsteroidal anti-inflammatory medicines (NSAIDs), as well as other medications, have been shown to aggravate IBS symptoms in some individuals and even cause them in others.

Changes in routine: Symptoms of irritable bowel syndrome may be triggered or made worse when there is a shift in a person's normal routine, such as when they go on vacation, start a new job, or their sleeping habits alter.

Infections: In some individuals, the beginning symptoms of irritable bowel syndrome (IBS) may be triggered by certain bacterial or viral illnesses of the stomach, such as gastroenteritis.

Physical activity: Extreme physical activity or exercise may bring on symptoms of irritable bowel syndrome (IBS) in some individuals, especially if the activity includes high impact or abdominal motions. Physical activity and exercise

It is essential to keep in mind that not all persons who have irritable bowel syndrome (IBS) have the same triggers, and it is even possible that some people may not have any identifiable triggers at all. Maintaining a food and symptom diary may help persons with irritable bowel syndrome (IBS)

discover personal triggers and provide them the ability to make adjustments in their diet or lifestyle in order to control their symptoms.

The part that stress and anxiety play in irritable bowel syndrome

It's well-accepted that worry and stress are major contributors to irritable bowel syndrome (IBS). According to the findings of some studies, up to sixty percent of persons who have irritable bowel syndrome also have a mental condition such as anxiety or depression. Although stress and worry are not thought to be the primary causes of irritable bowel syndrome (IBS), they may make symptoms worse and make it harder to control the condition.

Anxiety and stress may have a number of different effects on one's digestive system. For instance, they may enhance the motility of the gastrointestinal tract, which may result in stomach discomfort or diarrhea. They have also been shown to promote visceral hypersensitivity, which may make persons with irritable bowel syndrome more sensitive to pain and discomfort in the gastrointestinal tract. In addition, stress and worry may cause the body to go into a "fight or flight" reaction, which can result in the production of stress hormones such as cortisol and adrenaline. This can be a vicious cycle. These hormones may have an effect on the digestive tract by lowering blood flow to the intestines and causing the digestive process to go more slowly.

The management of stress and anxiety is an essential component in the management of symptoms associated with IBS. Taking slow, deep breaths, meditating, practicing yoga, and engaging in cognitive-behavioral therapy (also known as CBT) might be beneficial in lowering one's stress and anxiety levels. The use of stress management methods, such as biofeedback or relaxation treatment, may also be beneficial to some persons who have irritable bowel syndrome (IBS). While managing mental problems and improving IBS symptoms at the same time might be challenging, a doctor may decide to give medication, such as antidepressants or anti-anxiety drugs.

Research has indicated that stress and anxiety may have an effect on the microbiota of the gut, which may contribute to the symptoms of irritable bowel syndrome (IBS). The bacteria that reside in the gut and contribute to digestion, immunological function, and general health are collectively referred to as the gut microbiome. There are billions of microorganisms in the gut. The makeup and function of the gut microbiome may be altered by stress and anxiety, which can result in gut dysbiosis, also known as an imbalance of beneficial and harmful bacteria in the digestive tract. This may cause inflammation and immunological activation in the stomach, both of which may contribute to the symptoms of irritable bowel syndrome (IBS).

In addition, worry and stress have the potential to have an effect on the brain-gut axis, which is the communication network that exists between the stomach and the brain. This network is made up of a number of different components, one of which is called the enteric nervous system (ENS). The ENS is a network of neurons that controls digestive function and interacts with the central nervous system (CNS) through the vagus nerve. Stress and anxiety may disrupt this communication network, resulting in alterations in gastrointestinal motility, secretion, and sensitivity.

In general, stress and worry are multifaceted elements that may contribute to irritable bowel syndrome symptoms in a variety of different ways. The efficient management of stress and anxiety via a variety of strategies and treatments may be one of the most helpful ways to improve IBS symptoms and one's quality of life in general.

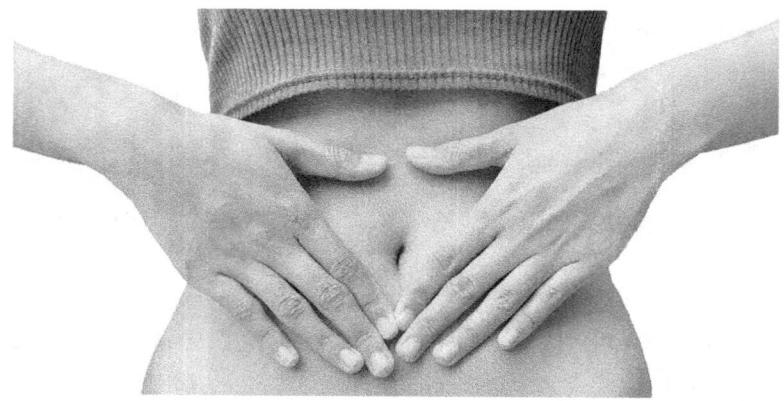

CHAPTER FOUR

Types of IBS

There are three primary forms of irritable bowel syndrome (IBS), which may be categorized according to the major bowel behaviors that a person experiences:

IBS with constipation (IBS-C)

Constipation is the primary symptom of a variant of irritable bowel syndrome known as IBS-C (irritable bowel syndrome with constipation). Individuals who suffer from IBS-C often have fewer than three bowel movements each week, on average. This is a typical symptom. They seldom have bowel movements, and when they do, the feces that they pass are often dry, hard, and difficult to pass. In addition to this, they could also feel bloating, discomfort, and stomach pain.

It is not entirely known what causes IBS-C; however, it is thought to be connected to irregularities in the way the muscles of the digestive system contract and relax. The specific etiology of IBS-C is not fully understood. Because of this, you may get constipation as a consequence of a delay in the transit of feces through the colon.

Those who have IBS-C may suffer various symptoms in addition to constipation. Some of these symptoms include:

- Straining during bowel movements
- A feeling of incomplete evacuation after a bowel movement
- Abdominal pain or discomfort
- Bloating or gas
- Mucus in the stool
- Nausea

Treatment: Changing one's food, making some adjustments to one's lifestyle, and maybe taking some medications are all common components of IBS-C treatment. Consuming foods that are high in fiber and drinking more water will assist to make stools easier to pass and encourage regular bowel motions. In addition to regular exercise and practices for stress reduction, getting enough sleep and being active may also help minimize symptoms. Laxatives, stool softeners, and prokinetic agents are some examples of the types of medications that a doctor could give in order to assist alleviate constipation and enhance bowel function.

IBS with diarrhea (IBS-D)

Irritable bowel syndrome with diarrhea, often known as IBS-D, is a variant of IBS in which diarrhea is the primary symptom. Individuals who suffer from IBS-D often have stools that are runny and loose, and they may have them more often than is customary. In addition to this, they can feel the need to have a bowel movement right afterward and have trouble keeping control of their bowel motions.

It is not entirely clear what causes irritable bowel syndrome with diarrhea (IBS-D), but one theory suggests that it is connected to changes in the way the muscles of the digestive system contract and relax. This may lead to an overactive colon, which can transport stool through the digestive system too rapidly, resulting in diarrhea. An underactive colon can have the opposite effect.

Those who have IBS-D may, in addition to experiencing diarrhea, also suffer from a variety of other symptoms, including the following:

• Abdominal pain or discomfort

• Bloating or gas

• Nausea

• Fatigue

- Urgency to have a bowel movement

- Incontinence or leakage of stool

Treatment

Modifications to one's diet and lifestyle, together with the use of medication, are commonly used to treat irritable bowel syndrome with diarrhea (IBS-D). Diets low in FODMAPs and avoiding foods that act as triggers are two strategies that may help minimize diarrhea and other symptoms. In order to assist improve the balance of bacteria in the stomach, your doctor may also prescribe taking probiotics. Antidiarrheal drugs, antispasmodics, and tricyclic antidepressants are some examples of the types of medications that a doctor could give to assist treat diarrhea as well as other symptoms. Methods for relieving stress and engaging in regular physical activity are both beneficial in this regard.

Mixed-type IBS (IBS-M)

Those who suffer from irritable bowel syndrome (IBS) may have a form known as Mixed-type IBS (IBS-M), in which they experience both constipation and diarrhea. This indicates that they may have loose stools one day and hard stools the next, or they may have a combination of both kinds of stools in a single bowel movement. Moreover, they may have a mixture of both types of feces at the same time. Individuals who suffer from IBS-M are more likely to encounter additional symptoms, including stomach pain or discomfort, bloating, and gas.

It is not completely known what causes IBS-M; however, it is thought to be connected to irregularities in the way the muscles of the digestive system contract and relax. The specific etiology of IBS-M is not entirely understood. Because of this, you could have bouts of constipation and diarrhea one after the other.

Those who have IBS-M are more likely to suffer the following symptoms in addition to constipation and diarrhea:

• Abdominal pain or discomfort

• Bloating or gas

• Nausea

• Fatigue

• Urgency to have a bowel movement

• Incontinence or leakage of stool

Medications, changes to the patient's food and lifestyle, and other behavioral and lifestyle adjustments are often included in the treatment plan for IBS-M. In order to alleviate symptoms, a nutritionist could suggest following a low-FODMAP diet or staying away from certain foods. In order to assist improve the balance of bacteria in the stomach, your doctor may also prescribe taking probiotics. Laxatives, antidiarrheal drugs, and antispasmodics are some examples of the types of medications that a doctor could give in order to assist regulate bowel function and alleviate symptoms. Methods for relieving stress and engaging in regular physical activity are both beneficial in this regard.

Symptoms And Characteristics of Each Type

Irritable bowel syndrome may be broken down into three distinct subcategories depending on the primary symptom that affects a person. The following is a list of symptoms and features that are associated with each form of IBS:

IBS with constipation (IBS-C)

- People who have IBS-C may also experience bloating, gas, abdominal pain or discomfort, and a feeling of incomplete evacuation after a bowel movement.

- Constipation is the primary symptom, which means having infrequent bowel movements or difficulty passing stools.
- Bowel movements may be hard, lumpy, or difficult to pass.

IBS with diarrhea (IBS-D)

- The most prominent symptom is diarrhea, which is characterized by passing stools that are loose and watery and that may take place more often than normal.
- Those who suffer from IBS-D are more likely to have symptoms such as an urgent need to defecate, stomach pain or discomfort, bloating, gas, and exhaustion.

Mixed-type IBS (IBS-M)

- Those who suffer from IBS-M often have both diarrhea and constipation.
- When a person has loose stools one time and hard stools the next time they have a bowel

movement, or when they have a bowel movement that contains both kinds of feces, they are said to have mixed stools.

- Those who suffer from IBS-M may also have stomach pain or discomfort, bloating, gas, and the sensation that they have not fully evacuated their bowels after a bowel movement.

It is essential to keep in mind that not everyone fits neatly into one of these categories and that some individuals may suffer a mix of symptoms that don't fit into any one subtype. It is also possible for people to have symptoms that do not fit into any of these subtypes. Those who suffer from irritable bowel syndrome often also struggle with other symptoms, including nausea, exhaustion, and urinary issues. The intensity of the symptoms and the frequency with which they appear may vary from person to person and may be affected by a variety of variables, including nutrition, stress, and changes in hormone levels.

The Diagnosis and Treatment Methods for Each Variant

It is possible for the diagnosis and therapy of each form of irritable bowel syndrome (IBS) to differ for each individual patient based on the symptoms they experience. Nonetheless, the following is a list of some of the most prevalent treatments for each form of IBS:

IBS with constipation (IBS-C)
Diagnosis:

- Before making a diagnosis, a physician would likely do a physical exam, go over the patient's medical history, and run tests to exclude other possible causes.
- They may use the Rome IV criteria to diagnose IBS-C, which includes having

recurrent abdominal pain on average at least one day per week in the last three months associated with two or more of the following: improved with defecation, onset associated with a change in frequency of stool, and onset associated with a change in form (appearance) of stool.

Treatment: In order to relieve symptoms, treatment consists of the following:

- A doctor may suggest modifications to the patient's lifestyle, including greater physical activity, a diet high in fiber, and increased water consumption.
- They could also recommend over-the-counter laxatives or drugs that need a prescription in order to alleviate the symptoms of constipation.

- There is some evidence that behavioral treatments, including cognitive behavioral therapy (CBT) and relaxation methods, may be beneficial in the treatment of symptoms.

IBS with diarrhea (IBS-D)

Diagnosis:

- The Rome IV criteria may be used by medical professionals in order to make a diagnosis of IBS-D, as was previously explained.
- They may also do tests to exclude the possibility of other diseases, such as inflammatory bowel disease (IBD).

Treatment:

- The treatment consists of making modifications to the patient's lifestyle, such as decreasing their level of stress, increasing the amount of physical exercise they get, and avoiding foods that trigger their symptoms.

- In certain cases, antidiarrheal medicines or bile acid binders are the treatments that doctors would provide to their patients in order to stop diarrhea.
- A doctor may also provide antibiotics or probiotics to assist with the regulation of bacteria found in the stomach.

Mixed-type IBS (IBS-M)

Diagnosis:

- The Rome IV criteria may be used by medical professionals in order to make a diagnosis of IBS-M, as was previously explained.
- They could also do testing to exclude the possibility of other disorders.

Treatment:

- The therapy for irritable bowel syndrome with constipation (IBS-C) and diarrhea (IBS-D) may be combined.
- Your doctor may recommend making adjustments to your lifestyle, such as increasing your fiber consumption, drinking more water, and avoiding foods that set off your symptoms.
- In order to control bowel movements, your doctor may recommend that you take medication such as laxatives or antidiarrheal medicines.
- Probiotics may also be suggested to help restore a healthy balance of bacteria in the gut and alleviate symptoms.

It is essential to keep in mind that a treatment strategy tailored specifically to an individual's unique set of symptoms and medical history may be required for that person. The treatment could potentially comprise a number of different treatments working together to treat a variety of symptoms.

CHAPTER FIVE

Diagnosing IBS

It may be difficult to diagnose irritable bowel syndrome (IBS) since the symptoms can range considerably and often overlap with those of other gastrointestinal conditions. On the other hand, healthcare professionals may diagnose IBS using any one of a number of different diagnostic tests. These are the following:

Detailed medical history and a complete physical exam: Your medical history will be reviewed, and your healthcare practitioner will ask you questions about your symptoms, including the frequency and intensity of stomach discomfort, bowel movements, and any other digestive symptoms you may be experiencing. They may also carry out a physical examination in order to look for any telltale symptoms of infection, inflammation, or any other hidden illnesses.

Rome IV Criteria: Irritable bowel syndrome (IBS) may be diagnosed using a set of recommendations known as the Rome IV Criteria. According to these criteria, a person must have recurrent abdominal pain on average at least one day per week in the last three months associated with two or more of the following: improved with defecation; onset associated with a change in frequency of stool; and onset associated with a change in form (appearance) of stool. In order to be diagnosed with IBS, a person must have had recurrent abdominal pain on average at least one day per week in the last three months.

Laboratory studies: In order to rule out other diseases, such as inflammatory bowel disease (IBD), celiac disease, or lactose intolerance, your healthcare professional may do tests on your blood, feces, or breath in the laboratory.

Endoscopic procedures: Endoscopy is a treatment that provides a healthcare professional with the ability to inspect the inside of a patient's digestive system. This method involves inserting a thin, flexible tube with a camera via the mouth or the rectum into the digestive system in order to observe the inside of the digestive tract. If the symptoms are severe or if they do not respond to therapy, this technique may be considered a diagnostic tool to help rule out other possible illnesses.

Irritable bowel syndrome (IBS) is a diagnostic of exclusion, which means that in order to diagnose IBS, one must first rule out the possibility of having another ailment that might be causing similar symptoms. Your primary care physician may also utilize additional diagnostic techniques or send you to a gastroenterologist (a physician who specializes in the diagnosis and treatment of digestive diseases) for further examination and management of your condition.

The Crucial Role of Eliminating All Other Possible Causes

Since many of these disorders need a different course of therapy than IBS does, it is crucial to rule out other conditions that could be generating symptoms that are similar to those caused by IBS. The following are some illnesses that may cause symptoms similar to those of IBS:

Inflammatory bowel disease (IBD): is a chronic inflammatory illness of the digestive system that encompasses Crohn's disease and ulcerative colitis. IBD is an abbreviation for inflammatory bowel disease. Abdominal discomfort, diarrhea, and bleeding from the rectal area are all possible symptoms of inflammatory bowel disease (IBD).

Celiac disease: Celiac disease is a hereditary autoimmune ailment in which the ingestion of gluten sets off an immune response that causes damage to the small intestine. Celiac disease is passed down via families. It's possible that you'll have bloating, stomach discomfort, and diarrhea as symptoms.

Overgrowth of bacteria in the small intestine, often known as SIBO: Symptoms of SIBO, which may include stomach discomfort, bloating, and diarrhea, can be brought on by an overgrowth of bacteria in the small intestine, which is what brings on SIBO.

Colon cancer: Symptoms of colon cancer include abdominal discomfort, bloating, and changes in bowel movements. Colon cancer may also cause changes in bowel habits.

Endometriosis is a condition in which the tissue that normally lines the inside of the uterus grows outside of it. This condition can cause symptoms such as abdominal pain, bloating, and changes in bowel habits. Endometriosis is a condition in which the tissue that normally lines the inside of the uterus grows outside of it.

It is possible for healthcare practitioners to guarantee that patients with IBS get an accurate diagnosis and the proper therapy by first excluding the possibility of other diseases. Those who are afflicted with the ailment may find that this makes it easier to control their symptoms and enhances their overall quality of life.

A wide range of diagnostic procedures, such as the following examples, may be carried out by medical professionals in order to rule out other possible causes.

Tests on the blood: Tests on the blood may be done to look for indicators of inflammation, anemia, or other disorders that could be causing the symptoms that the patient is experiencing.

Tests performed on the stool: Stool tests are one method that may be used to screen for infections and other digestive system disorders.

Colonoscopy: A colonoscopy is a technique that involves looking into the interior of the colon with the use of a very tiny camera. During this operation, evidence of inflammation, polyps, and other abnormalities may be looked for in the patient's digestive tract.

Imaging testing: Imaging tests, such as CT scans or MRIs, may be performed to check for evidence of inflammation, obstructions, or other abnormalities in the digestive system.

Examples of these tests include the following:

Endoscopy is a medical technique that involves inspecting the inside of the digestive system with the use of a very tiny camera. During this treatment, symptoms of inflammation, ulcers, and other anomalies might be looked for if the patient so desires.

Irritable bowel syndrome (IBS) may be diagnosed using certain criteria when the possibility of other diseases has been eliminated. Irritable bowel syndrome (IBS) is often diagnosed by using the Rome criteria, which stipulate that the patient must have had stomach pain or discomfort on at least three days per month for at least three months, in addition to having two or more of the following symptoms:

- A reduction in the severity of symptoms after a bowel movement
- The beginning of symptoms associated with shifts in the regularity of bowel movements
- The beginning of symptoms associated with shifts in the consistency of stools

Irritable bowel syndrome may be effectively diagnosed and an effective treatment plan can be formulated for patients with the help of these criteria.

Tests To Diagnose Irritable Bowel Syndrome

There are no diagnostic tests that are unique to IBS; however, various tests may be done to rule out other disorders that can produce symptoms that are similar to those of IBS. In order to identify irritable bowel syndrome (IBS) and rule out other disorders, several of the following tests may be performed:

Tests on the blood: Tests on the blood may be done to look for evidence of infection or inflammation, as well as for anemia.

Tests performed on the stool: Tests performed on the stool may be used to look for evidence of infection or inflammation in the digestive tract.

Colonoscopy: A colonoscopy is a diagnostic procedure that involves examining the inside of the colon with the use of a long, flexible tube equipped with a camera. It is possible to utilize it to search for evidence of inflammation, polyps, or other abnormalities.

A flexible sigmoidoscopy is a diagnostic procedure that involves the utilization of a flexible tube that is fitted with a camera in order to inspect the interior of the lower portion of the colon. It is possible to utilize it to search for evidence of inflammation, polyps, or other abnormalities.

X-rays: X-rays are a diagnostic tool that can be used to examine the digestive tract for any blockages or other abnormalities.

Tests of the breath: Tests of the breath may be done to determine whether or not there is an excess of bacteria in the small intestine.

These tests are not used to diagnose irritable bowel syndrome (IBS), but rather to rule out other disorders that might be generating symptoms that are similar to those of IBS. This is a crucial point to keep in mind. The patient's symptoms, as well as their medical history and the outcomes of any diagnostic tests that were carried out, are often used to arrive at a diagnosis of irritable bowel syndrome (IBS).

CHAPTER SIX

Treatment Options for IBS

The therapy for irritable bowel syndrome (IBS) differs according to the intensity of the patient's symptoms as well as the kind of IBS they are experiencing. There are several different treatment options available for irritable bowel syndrome (IBS), including the following:

Alterations to one's diet: Altering one's diet may be able to help ease the symptoms of IBS. For instance, increasing fiber intake may help ease constipation in patients with irritable bowel syndrome type C, but decreasing fiber intake and avoiding trigger foods like coffee and alcohol may help lessen symptoms in patients with irritable bowel syndrome type D.

Medication: There are a number of medications that can be used to treat the symptoms of irritable bowel syndrome. These medications include antispasmodics, which are used to treat abdominal pain, laxatives, which are used to treat constipation, and anti-diarrheal medications, which are used to treat diarrhea.

Psychological treatments: Cognitive-behavioral therapy (CBT) and hypnotherapy are two examples of psychological therapies that have the potential to be beneficial in the management of IBS symptoms, particularly those symptoms that are associated with stress and anxiety.

Probiotics: Probiotics, which are helpful bacteria that dwell in the gut, may help ease the symptoms of irritable bowel syndrome (IBS) by restoring the balance of the bacteria that live in the gut.

Regular exercise: may assist improve bowel function and decrease stress, both of which may contribute to the symptoms of IBS. Exercise may also help lower the risk of developing IBS.

Alternative treatments: Some patients find that using alternative treatments, such as acupuncture and herbal medications, is beneficial in treating the symptoms of irritable bowel syndrome (IBS).

It is essential to keep in mind that there is no cure-all therapy for irritable bowel syndrome (IBS) and that a medication that helps one person may not help another. Finding the treatment method that works best for a person who has IBS may need some trial and error on the part of the patient. Also, it is essential to have a tight working relationship with a healthcare practitioner in order to regularly evaluate symptoms and make therapy adjustments as required.

Adapting Your Way of Life to Ease the Symptoms of Irritable Bowel Syndrome

Alterations to one's lifestyle, in addition to the many therapy methods that were just discussed, may be of great assistance in the management of IBS symptoms. Changes in the following aspects of one's lifestyle may prove to be beneficial:

Management of stress: Since stress may bring on symptoms of irritable bowel syndrome (IBS), it might be useful to acquire skills for managing stress, such as deep breathing, meditation, yoga, or other relaxation techniques.

Exercise on a regular basis: Exercising on a regular basis may assist improve bowel function and decrease stress, both of which can help relieve symptoms of irritable bowel syndrome (IBS).

Sleep: Obtaining a sufficient amount of sleep is essential for maintaining general health, and research has shown that not getting enough sleep may make IBS symptoms worse. It is suggested that you get between seven and nine hours of sleep each night.

Avoid trigger foods: Some individuals have symptoms of irritable bowel syndrome (IBS) when they eat certain foods. It is essential to maintain a food diary in order to determine which foods are responsible for triggering symptoms and to thereafter abstain from eating those meals.

Eat smaller, more frequent meals: Have fewer, smaller meals more often While eating big meals might bring on IBS symptoms, consuming fewer, smaller meals more frequently can be helpful.

Stay away from tobacco products and drink alcohol in moderation: While smoking and drinking too much alcohol may both make IBS symptoms worse; it is advisable to avoid doing either of these things as much as possible.

Hydration: Maintaining proper hydration is essential for general health, and dehydration may make symptoms of irritable bowel syndrome (IBS) worse. At least eight full glasses of water should be consumed daily since this is what is suggested.

Intake of fiber: Although increasing the amount of fiber consumed might be beneficial for some individuals who have irritable bowel syndrome (IBS), it is necessary to do so gradually in order to prevent making symptoms worse. Particularly advantageous is the soluble fiber, which may be found in foods such as oats and beans, in addition to several fruits and vegetables.

Probiotics: There is evidence from some research to indicate that taking probiotics, which are live bacteria and yeasts that are good for the health of the digestive tract, may be useful in the treatment of IBS symptoms. Either in the form of fermented foods such as yogurt, kefir, sauerkraut, and kimchi or in the form of supplements, probiotics are abundant.

Eating consciously: Eating mindfully, also known as paying attention to your body's signs of hunger and fullness, may be useful for controlling the symptoms of irritable bowel syndrome (IBS). Eating slowly and carefully chewing food may also be beneficial, so keep that in mind.

Avoiding carbonated drinks: is highly recommended for those who have irritable bowel syndrome (IBS) since carbonated beverages are known to cause bloating and gas.

Heat therapy: Applying heat to the belly, such as with a heating pad or by taking a warm bath, may help ease the abdominal pain and discomfort associated with irritable bowel syndrome (IBS).

It is essential to keep in mind that not all adjustments in lifestyle will be beneficial for a person who has irritable bowel syndrome (IBS), and some may potentially make symptoms worse. It is in your best interest to engage with a healthcare expert to determine which modifications in lifestyle may be most useful for your particular symptoms and scenario.

Medicines that may treat IBS

The symptoms of irritable bowel syndrome (IBS) may be managed with the use of a number of different drugs. The following are examples of popular drugs used in the treatment of IBS:

Antispasmodics: are a kind of medication that helps ease the discomfort associated with stomach cramps. These medicines function by easing the tension in the muscles that line the intestinal tract. Hyoscyamine and dicyclomine are two examples of antispasmodics that are often used.

Laxatives: Laxatives are an option for treating constipation in those who suffer from IBS-C. There are many different kinds of laxatives available, such as osmotic laxatives, stimulant laxatives, and stool softeners. Osmotic laxatives are the most common form.

Antidiarrheals: Antidiarrheals are a treatment option for diarrhea in those who suffer from IBS-D. These drugs are effective because they reduce the rate of movement of the bowels.

Antidiarrheals such as loperamide and diphenoxylate/atropine are often used.

Supplements with fiber: Those who suffer from IBS-C and constipation may get relief from constipation by taking fiber supplements. The way that these supplements operate is by increasing the weight of the stool, which in turn makes it easier for the feces to pass through the intestines. Psyllium and methylcellulose are two examples of fiber supplements that are available.

Probiotics: The term "probiotics" refers to living bacteria and yeasts that are useful to the health of the digestive tract. According to the findings of certain research, using probiotics may be of assistance in the treatment of IBS symptoms.

Low-dose antidepressants: irritable bowel syndrome (IBS) may cause abdominal pain and discomfort, both of which can be treated with low-dose tricyclic antidepressants (TCAs) and selective serotonin reuptake inhibitors (SSRIs). These drugs function by modifying the amounts of certain neurotransmitters in the stomach in order to achieve their desired effects.

Cognitive behavioral therapy (CBT): is a sort of treatment that may assist individuals who suffer from irritable bowel syndrome (IBS) in better-managing stress and anxiety, both of which can make symptoms worse.

Hypnotherapy: is a sort of treatment that may be helpful in the management of symptoms of irritable bowel syndrome (IBS), especially for people who suffer from IBS-D.

Acupuncture: is a kind of alternative medicine that involves inserting very tiny needles into various sites all over the body. There is evidence from a few trials to indicate that acupuncture may be useful in the treatment of IBS symptoms.

Peppermint oil: Peppermint oil is a natural product that has the potential to help alleviate the symptoms of irritable bowel syndrome (IBS). The muscles in the intestines are relaxed, which allows them to operate, and inflammation is also reduced.

Diet of elimination: in order to determine whether or not certain foods are responsible for causing your symptoms, an elimination diet requires that you cut out specific items from your diet. Dairy products, wheat, and even certain kinds of fruits and vegetables might be foods that bring on symptoms of irritable bowel syndrome (IBS).

It is essential to keep in mind that not all of these therapies will help people who have irritable bowel syndrome (IBS), and some of them may potentially make symptoms worse. It is in your best interest to collaborate with a healthcare expert in order to determine which therapies have the potential to be the most useful for your particular set of symptoms and circumstances.

Alternate treatments for irritable bowel syndrome

The symptoms of irritable bowel syndrome (IBS) have led researchers to investigate a number of different alternative treatments. It is crucial to highlight that there is minimal scientific evidence to support the usefulness of these treatments, even if there is a possibility that some individuals may find them beneficial. The following are some examples of alternative treatments for IBS:

Probiotics: Supplements containing probiotic bacteria, which are helpful microorganisms that may assist enhance digestive health, are known as probiotics. Probiotics have shown promise in a number of trials as a potential treatment for irritable bowel syndrome (IBS), especially in patients diagnosed with IBS-D.

Herbal remedies: It's possible that peppermint, ginger, and fennel, among other herbs, might help lessen the symptoms of irritable bowel syndrome (IBS). Nevertheless, before taking any herbal therapies, it is essential to see a healthcare expert, since herbal medicines may combine with other prescriptions or make symptoms worse.

Massage treatment: Studies have shown that massage therapy may help decrease tension and anxiety, both of which can make symptoms of irritable bowel syndrome (IBS) worse.

Meditation and yoga: Regularly practicing meditation and yoga may help decrease stress and anxiety, which in turn may make it easier to manage the symptoms of IBS.

Aromatherapy: Aromatherapy, also known as essential oil treatment, is the use of aromatic plant oils to treat stress and induce relaxation. There is some evidence that some essential oils, such as peppermint and lavender, may help alleviate the symptoms of irritable bowel syndrome (IBS).

When it comes to the management of IBS symptoms, it is always preferable to work with a healthcare professional to build a thorough treatment plan. It is crucial to keep in mind that alternative treatments should not be used as a replacement for conventional medical therapy.

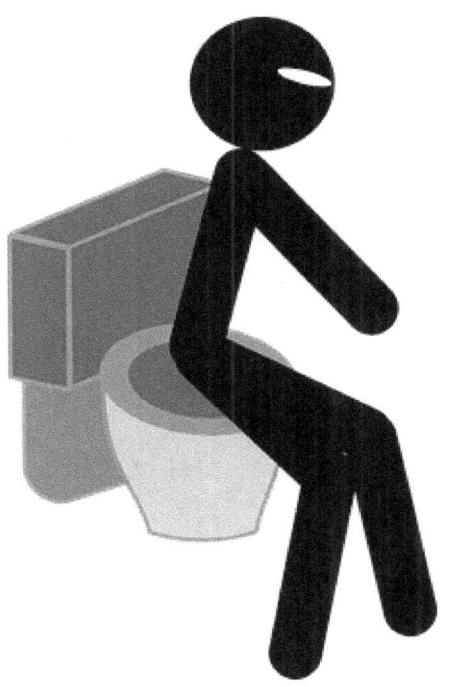

CHAPTER SEVEN

Diet and Nutrition for IBS

Food and nutrition play a significant part in the management of symptoms associated with IBS. Although no one treatment is guaranteed to work for everyone, making some adjustments to one's diet may be beneficial in the management of symptoms. The following is a list of dietary advice for the management of IBS:

Keep a record of what you eat: Maintain a record of the meals you consume and how your symptoms change as a result of those foods. This information may assist you in determining the items that cause your reaction and in making the appropriate adjustments to your diet.

Eat smaller, more frequent meals: Consuming meals that are smaller in size but are consumed more often during the day may alleviate symptoms such as bloating, gas, and stomach discomfort.

Avoid trigger foods: Avoid eating things that may set off your IBS symptoms, such as fatty or fried meals, dairy products, chocolate, caffeine, alcohol, and fizzy drinks. You should probably stay away from meals that contain a lot of sugar or fiber as well.

Increase fiber intake: It may be helpful for some individuals who have irritable bowel syndrome (IBS) to increase their fiber intake; however, it is essential to do so in a progressive manner to prevent making symptoms worse. In general, foods strong in soluble fiber, like oatmeal, bananas, and berries, are simpler to digest than meals high in insoluble fiber, such as wheat bran and raw fruits and vegetables. Soluble fiber is found in foods like oatmeal, bananas, and berries.

Stay hydrated: Maintaining proper hydration by consuming a sufficient amount of water at regular intervals throughout the day will assist in warding off constipation and maintaining proper hydration.

Consider a low FODMAP diet: Try following a diet low in fermentable oligosaccharides, disaccharides, and polyols (low FODMAP). The low FODMAP diet is a specific diet that is aimed to minimize the intake of particular kinds of carbohydrates that may contribute to the symptoms of irritable bowel syndrome (IBS). To make sure that you are getting the proper amount of nutrients while following this diet, you should seek the advice of a qualified dietitian or a healthcare expert.

Keep in mind that the requirements of everyone's diet are varied and that what works well for one person may not work well for another. When it comes to developing a specific dietary plan for the management of IBS symptoms, it is important to collaborate with a healthcare physician or a registered dietitian.

The Importance of Food in the Treatment of IBS

Nutrition is an extremely important component in the treatment of irritable bowel syndrome (IBS). Some meals and drinks might bring on irritable bowel syndrome symptoms such as bloating, stomach discomfort, constipation, and diarrhea, even if the actual etiology of the condition is unknown. Irritable bowel syndrome (IBS) cannot be treated with a universally effective diet, and dietary suggestions must be adapted to each person.

IBS symptoms may be managed, however, by following a few fundamental dietary rules.

The low FODMAP diet is one kind of eating plan that has garnered a lot of attention as a potential treatment for irritable bowel syndrome (IBS). Carbohydrates known as FODMAPs (fermentable oligosaccharides, disaccharides, monosaccharides, and polyols) may be poorly absorbed in the small intestine and may be a factor in the development of symptoms associated with irritable bowel syndrome (IBS). Restricting high-FODMAP foods and then gradually returning them as part of the low-FODMAP diet is one way to narrow down the list of items that are causing symptoms.

Other dietary advice for the management of IBS symptoms includes the following:

- o Consuming fewer, smaller meals throughout the day to avoid bloating and stomach pain.

- Consuming a large amount of water to maintain proper hydration and avoid developing constipation.
- Staying away from meals that may set off your allergic reaction, such as those high in caffeine or fat, as well as alcohol and spices.
- Increase the amount of fiber that you consume, whether via food or supplements, to treat constipation. Yet, some individuals who have IBS can benefit from reducing the amount of fiber they consume.
- Consuming a well-rounded diet that is comprised of a variety of foods, including fruits, vegetables, grains, and proteins that are low in fat.

When it comes to developing a specific dietary plan for the management of IBS symptoms, it is important to collaborate with a healthcare physician or a registered dietitian. They can assist in the identification of foods that cause reactions and provide dietary advice based on the individual's requirements and preferences.

In addition to the basic dietary guidelines, there are some items that, depending on the person, may be helpful or detrimental for those who have irritable bowel syndrome (IBS):

Foods that are good for you:

Probiotics: These are living microorganisms that have the potential to promote digestive health and lower inflammatory responses. Yogurt, kefir, kimchi, sauerkraut, and kombucha are examples of foods that are high in probiotics.

Low-FODMAP meals: are also beneficial since, as was noted previously, some carbs may cause IBS symptoms. Rice, quinoa, oats, potatoes, carrots, cucumbers, grapes, oranges, strawberries, and lactose-free dairy products are examples of foods that fall into the low-FODMAP category.

Peppermint: This plant, peppermint, contains antispasmodic effects that may help decrease belly discomfort and bloating. Peppermint is a popular digestive aid. Tea or supplements containing peppermint may be helpful for some people who suffer from irritable bowel syndrome (IBS).

Harmful foods:

High-FODMAP foods: Foods that are high in FODMAPs include wheat, rye, and barley as well as onions, garlic, apples, pears, honey, and high-fructose corn syrup. Other foods that are high in FODMAPs include onions, garlic, and onions.

Gas-producing foods: Foods that cause gas Some foods, such as beans, lentils, and cruciferous vegetables (broccoli, cauliflower, and cabbage), may contribute to bloating and discomfort by creating gas.

Fried and fatty foods: Fried meals and foods high in fat may be difficult to digest, which can make diarrhea worse for certain people who suffer from irritable bowel syndrome (IBS).

It is essential to keep in mind that people have varying levels of tolerance for various kinds of food and that what works for one person may not work for another. Maintaining a food diary and keeping track of symptoms may help identify items that may act as triggers and in developing an appropriate diet plan.

Foods That Should Be Avoided and Foods That Should Be Included

It is essential for people who have irritable bowel syndrome (IBS) to emphasize meals that are simple to digest and less likely to bring on symptoms. The following is a list of some general dietary recommendations:

Foods to steer clear of:

High-FODMAP foods: Foods high in fermentable oligosaccharides, polyols, and monosaccharides are carbohydrates that are poorly absorbed in the small intestine and are known to produce bloating and gas. Wheat, rye, barley, onions, garlic, apples, pears, honey, and high-fructose corn syrup are some examples of foods that contain gluten.

Gas-producing foods: Foods that cause gas Some foods, such as beans, lentils, and cruciferous vegetables (broccoli, cauliflower, and cabbage), may contribute to bloating and discomfort by creating gas.

Caffeine and alcohol: Both caffeine and alcohol have been shown to stimulate the digestive tract, which may make diarrhea worse in certain people.

Fried and fatty foods: Fried meals and foods high in fat may be difficult to digest, which can make diarrhea worse for certain people who suffer from irritable bowel syndrome (IBS).

Foods to include

Low-FODMAP foods: These are carbohydrates that are easily digested and less likely to cause symptoms. Examples include rice, quinoa, oats, potatoes, carrots, cucumbers, grapes, oranges, strawberries, and lactose-free dairy products.

Soluble fiber: This form of fiber, known as soluble fiber, is beneficial for regulating bowel motions and relieving constipation. Oats, barley, and psyllium are examples of foods that are high in soluble fiber.

Soluble fiber may also be found in fruits like bananas, apples, and berries.

Lean protein: Proteins found in lean meats such as chicken, fish, tofu, and eggs are excellent sources of protein that are simple to digest and less prone to induce symptoms.

Fats that are good for you: Olive oil, avocados, nuts, and seeds are all examples of foods that contain healthy fats and may offer energy without making symptoms worse.

It is essential to keep in mind that people have varying levels of tolerance for various kinds of food and that what works for one person may not work for another. Maintaining a food diary and keeping track of symptoms may help identify items that may act as triggers and in developing an appropriate diet plan. When designing a specific meal plan for the treatment of IBS, seeking the advice of a licensed dietitian might be another beneficial strategy.

Special diets for IBS, such as the low FODMAP diet The low FODMAP diet is a common and successful dietary strategy for the management of symptoms associated with IBS. Those who suffer from irritable bowel syndrome (IBS) are more likely to have digestive symptoms such as bloating, gas, and diarrhea as a result of their inability to properly absorb certain carbohydrates known as FODMAPs. The low FODMAP diet involves avoiding or limiting high-FODMAP foods for some time, typically two to six weeks, and then reintroducing them one by one to determine which ones cause symptoms. Symptoms can be caused by foods that contain fermentable small oligosaccharides (FODMAPS), which are found in fruits and vegetables. The following are some examples of foods that are considered to be high in FODMAP:

- Wheat and other gluten-containing grains
- Dairy products
- Certain fruits, such as apples, peaches, and mangoes
- Certain vegetables, such as onions, garlic, and mushrooms
- Legumes, such as beans and lentils
- Sweeteners, such as honey and agave nectar

It is essential to substitute items that are high in FODMAPs with alternatives that are low in FODMAPs when following the elimination phase of the low FODMAP diet. This will ensure that the diet remains well-balanced and healthy. The following are some examples of foods that are low on the FODMAP scale:

- Gluten-free grains, such as rice, quinoa, and oats.
- Lactose-free dairy products or non-dairy alternatives, such as almond milk.

- Low-FODMAP fruits, such as strawberries, blueberries, and grapes.
- Low-FODMAP vegetables, such as carrots, spinach, and bell peppers.
- Protein sources, such as meat, fish, eggs, and tofu.
- Nuts and seeds, such as almonds and pumpkin seeds.

To alleviate the discomfort associated with irritable bowel syndrome (IBS), many people turn to a particular diet known as the low FODMAP diet. FODMAPs are short-chain carbohydrates that are poorly absorbed in the small intestine. This causes digestive discomfort in certain individuals, especially those who have irritable bowel syndrome (IBS).

The low FODMAP diet is cutting down on foods that are rich in FODMAPs for a certain amount of time, often between four and six weeks, and then gradually reintroducing those foods to figure out which one's cause symptoms. The goal is to find a way to limit FODMAP consumption to alleviate symptoms while still consuming a diet that is rich in variety and well-balanced to get the right amount of essential nutrients.

Some fruits and vegetables, including apples, pears, and melons; certain legumes, including beans, lentils, and chickpeas; wheat and other gluten-containing grains; and Sweeteners such as honey, agave, and high fructose corn syrups are some of the items that are not allowed on a low FODMAP diet.

- Meats, fish, and poultry
- Eggs
- Rice, quinoa, and other gluten-free grains
- Most vegetables, including carrots, zucchini, and spinach
- Most fruits, including bananas, grapes, and oranges

- Lactose-free dairy products, such as lactose-free milk and cheese substitutes
- Certain nuts and seeds, such as almonds and chia seeds

Since it may be challenging to stick to and may lead to nutritional shortages if it is not followed correctly, the low FODMAP diet should only be taken under the supervision of a qualified medical expert. This is an essential point to keep in mind, as it is crucial to highlight. It is essential to reintroduce foods progressively containing FODMAPs, since some individuals may be able to handle tiny quantities without bringing on symptoms even if they have IBS.

CHAPTER EIGHT

Coping with IBS

Dealing with irritable bowel syndrome (IBS) may be difficult, particularly if the symptoms are severe and interfere with everyday living. The following is a list of suggestions for managing with IBS:

Maintain your vigilance: Get as much information as you can on irritable bowel syndrome and the things that bring on your symptoms. Having this information may assist you in better understanding your illness and efficiently managing the symptoms you are experiencing.

Maintain a log of your symptoms: Maintaining a journal of your symptoms might assist you in determining trends as well as causes. Keep a journal of everything you eat, how you feel, and anything else you can think of that could be causing or contributing to your symptoms.

Practice stress reduction techniques: irritable bowel syndrome (IBS) symptoms may be made worse by stress; therefore, it is important to find effective ways to decrease your level of anxiety and tension. You may control your symptoms and experience less stress with the use of stress relief techniques like meditation, deep breathing, yoga, and exercise.

Get support: Communicating about the emotional burden of living with IBS with friends, family, or a therapist might help you learn to control those feelings. Moreover, support groups are a great resource for both knowledge and emotional assistance.

Be patient: It may take some time to find an appropriate therapy and method for managing symptoms, so be patient and persistent in your attempts to find these things.

Maintain a positive outlook: Living with irritable bowel syndrome (IBS) may be tough at times, but putting your attention on the activities and pursuits that bring you the most pleasure and satisfaction will help you keep a good attitude and enhance the quality of your life.

Always try to have a healthy lifestyle: To alleviate the symptoms of irritable bowel syndrome (IBS) and improve one's overall health and well-being, it is essential to maintain a healthy diet, engage in regular physical activity, and receive an adequate amount of sleep.

Methods for Taking Control of One's Anxiety and Stress

The following is a list of techniques that may be of use in the management of stress and anxiety related to IBS:

Meditation on mindfulness: Regular practice of meditation on mindfulness may assist you in being more aware of your thoughts and emotions, as well as in cultivating a stronger sense of peace and relaxation in your body and mind. This may be particularly useful in lowering the tension and anxiety that are linked with irritable bowel syndrome (IBS).

Exercise: Frequent exercise may help to ease some of the symptoms of irritable bowel syndrome (IBS), including tension and anxiety, and it can also help to minimize the risk of developing IBS. Try to complete at least half an hour of moderate-intensity physical activity on most days of the week.

Techniques of relaxation: There are a variety of relaxation methods that may be beneficial for managing the tension and anxiety associated with irritable bowel syndrome (IBS). Some examples of these techniques include deep breathing, progressive muscle relaxation, and guided imagery.

Cognitive-behavioral treatment, sometimes referred to as CBT: The primary goals of cognitive behavioral therapy (CBT), a kind of talk therapy, are to recognize and alter destructive patterns of behavior and cognition. Particularly useful for the management of stress and anxiety linked with irritable bowel syndrome (IBS), it may be.

Support groups: Participating in a support group designed specifically for individuals who have irritable bowel syndrome (IBS) may be a beneficial method to connect with others who are going through symptoms that are comparable to your own as well as to learn coping skills from other people.

Time management: Feeling overloaded or unorganized might be a contributing factor in the development of stress. Time management and stress reduction may both benefit from the creation of a timetable or list of things to accomplish.

Self-care: Take care of yourself by participating in things that make you happy, such as pursuing a hobby or spending time with people you care about. It might assist reduce anxiety and tension.

Irritable Bowel Syndrome (IBS) Support Groups and Other Resources

Those who suffer from irritable bowel syndrome and are searching for information and assistance may choose from a wide variety of sites. Among the available choices are:

IBS support groups: Support groups for those who suffer from irritable bowel syndrome (IBS) may be found at several local hospitals and community organizations. Those who are going through difficulties comparable to their own might benefit from participating in these groups because they provide a forum in which they can discuss their situations, get answers to their queries, and network with others in a similar situation.

Online forums: People with IBS may interact with others from all over the globe by participating in one of the several online groups or forums that are specifically devoted to the condition. Irritable

Bowel Syndrome Network, the Irritable Bowel Syndrome Association, and the IBS community on Reddit are three popular choices.

Educational resources: There are many educational materials available, such as books, websites, and online courses, which give information about irritable bowel syndrome (IBS) and how to treat it. The low FODMAP diet app developed by Monash University, the website of the International Foundation for Gastrointestinal Diseases, and the book Gut Health Diet for Beginners written by Gabriela Gardner are just a few of the popular resources available.

Counseling and psychotherapy: The psychological side of IBS may be difficult to manage for some individuals, and this can be a challenge for them. Developing techniques for managing IBS and lowering stress and anxiety may both benefit from seeing a therapist or counselor who specializes in treating IBS.

Those who specialize in nutrition and dietetics: If you have irritable bowel syndrome (IBS), it may be useful to work with a registered dietitian who specializes in IBS to establish a personalized diet plan that is tailored to match the requirements and preferences of the individual.

Apps: Those who suffer from IBS have access to some helpful applications that may assist with keeping track of their symptoms, dietary consumption, and stress levels. Cara Care, MySymptoms Food Diary, and Bowelle are three solutions that do rather well in the market.

The International Foundation for Gastrointestinal Disorders (IFFGD): is a charitable organization that was established with the mission of assisting those who suffer from gastrointestinal conditions. Those who suffer from irritable bowel syndrome may turn to them for information, resources, and support.

National Institute of Diabetes and Digestive and Kidney Diseases (NIDDK): People who are afflicted by digestive problems, such as irritable bowel syndrome (IBS), have access to a wealth of information and services thanks to the National Institute of Diabetes and Digestive and Kidney Diseases (NIDDK), which is a division of the National Institutes of Health (NIH).

Crohn's and Colitis Foundation: Those who have irritable bowel syndrome (IBS) and persons who have other inflammatory bowel disorders may get support and information from the Crohn's and Colitis Foundation, which is a charitable organization.

Online support groups: Support groups and forums available online There are some support groups and forums available online for people who have irritable bowel syndrome (IBS), where people can talk about their experiences, ask questions, and get support from others who are going through experiences that are similar to their own.

Professionals in the healthcare industry: Those who suffer from irritable bowel syndrome and are searching for additional direction on how to manage their symptoms may find it beneficial to seek the advice of a healthcare expert, such as a gastroenterologist or a certified dietitian.

Advice on coping with the symptoms of IBS

It may be difficult to live with irritable bowel syndrome (IBS), but there are some techniques and approaches that can assist people in managing their symptoms and improving their quality of life. The following are some of these pointers:

Maintain a log of your symptoms: Keeping a journal of your symptoms, what you ate, and how you felt might help determine trends and identify triggers.

Plan: While going out in public, it is important to do some planning to determine where the toilets are and to pack any essential prescriptions or supplies for special dietary requirements.

Participate in Activities That Help You Relax: Irritable bowel syndrome (IBS) symptoms may be made worse by stress, therefore it's important to practice relaxation methods like deep breathing and meditation.

Exercise regularly: Frequent exercise may help regulate bowel motions and decrease stress, so it's important to make sure you're getting enough of it.

Stay hydrated: Maintaining enough hydration by drinking a lot of water may help avoid constipation and maintain the health of the digestive tract.

Obtain enough rest: Not only is sleep essential for general health, but it may also assist in the management of stress and the reduction of weariness.

Request support: Discuss your experiences with irritable bowel syndrome (IBS) with friends, relatives, or members of a support group. Reaching out for assistance may help reduce feelings of stress and worry.

Take control of your diet: Take charge of your nutrition by formulating, in collaboration with a trained medical practitioner, a meal plan that caters to both your preferences and the specific requirements of your body.

Do not disregard any symptoms: If symptoms become worse or shift, it is important to see a healthcare expert. It is essential to rule out any other possible disorders that may be present.

CHAPTER NINE

Future Directions in IBS Research and Treatment

Research on IBS has advanced significantly in recent years, and continuous attempts are being made to better understand the underlying causes of the condition and create novel therapies for it. The following is a list of some of the prospective areas of investigation and therapy for IBS:

The creation of brand-new pharmaceuticals: irritable bowel syndrome (IBS) is one of the most common digestive disorders, and scientists are always looking for novel ways to treat it, including developing drugs that target the microbiome and inflammation in the gut.

Precision medicine: There is a rising interest in the use of tailored techniques to treat IBS, depending on a patient's particular symptoms, medical history, and genetic makeup. This area of medicine is referred to as "precision medicine."

Research on the gut-brain axis: Scientists are now investigating the intricate connection that exists between the stomach and the brain, in the hopes of discovering novel ways to treat irritable bowel syndrome (IBS) and the underlying causes of the condition.

Interventions that do not involve the use of drugs: non-pharmacological approaches to the management of irritable bowel syndromes (IBS), such as cognitive-behavioral therapy, mindfulness-based stress reduction, and hypnotherapy, are garnering a growing amount of attention.

Patient-centered care: Care that is oriented toward the patient is becoming an increasingly important priority. This kind of care takes into consideration the specific requirements and inclinations of each patient and encourages them to take an active role in their medical treatment.

Ongoing education and awareness: It is necessary to conduct ongoing education and awareness initiatives to assist the general population in better comprehending IBS and lowering the stigma that is associated with the condition.

Those who suffer from irritable bowel syndrome (IBS) have reason to have optimism that as science continues to grow, new and improved therapies will be produced that will assist them in managing their symptoms and enhancing their quality of life.

The latest findings from studies on IBS

Research on IBS is now being conducted with a focus on a variety of topics, including the following:

Gut microbiome: irritable bowel syndrome (IBS) has been linked to changes in the microbiome of the gut, which has been the subject of research. Irritable bowel syndrome (IBS) is a common digestive disorder, and researchers are now looking into the possible links between gut bacteria and potential therapies that might target the gut microbiome.

Neurotransmitters: are substances that are released by nerve cells to allow for communication with other nerve cells. Recent research points to an imbalance in neurotransmitters as a possible factor in the development of irritable bowel syndrome (IBS). Ongoing studies are being conducted to better understand the function neurotransmitters play in irritable bowel syndrome (IBS) and to create novel medications that specifically target these neurotransmitters.

Genetics: Irritable bowel syndrome has been observed to run in families, which lends credence to the theory that genetics may play a part in the condition's onset. The identification of certain genes that could have a role in irritable bowel syndrome (IBS) by researchers might pave the way for the development of novel medicines for the condition.

Immune system: There is some speculation that the immune system is involved in the development of irritable bowel syndrome (IBS). Ongoing studies are being conducted to better understand the function that the immune system plays in irritable bowel syndrome (IBS) and to develop novel medicines that specifically target the immune system.

New treatments: Novel treatments are now being researched by medical professionals for irritable bowel syndrome (IBS). These new treatments include new drugs and therapies, such as cognitive behavioral therapy and hypnosis.

In general, the primary goals of ongoing research on irritable bowel syndrome (IBS) are to better understand the factors that contribute to the development of the illness and to come up with novel therapies that are both more successful and less severe than those that are now available.

Exciting Breakthrough Therapies on the Horizon for IBS

Some intriguing novel medicines are now under investigation for IBS. The following are some of the more noteworthy ones:

Microbial therapies: Researchers are looking at the possibility of treating irritable bowel syndrome using fecal microbiota transplantation (FMT) and other types of microbial therapies, which work by modifying the makeup of the microbiome found in the gut.

Serotonin receptor modulators: Modulators of serotonin receptors Serotonin is a neurotransmitter that works to regulate the sensitivity and motility of the gastrointestinal tract. By influencing the levels of serotonin in the gut, serotonin receptor modulators such as alosetron and tegaserod have shown some promise in lowering the symptoms of irritable bowel syndrome (IBS).

Immune modulators: Recent research has revealed that a disturbance in the immune system may play a role in the development of irritable bowel syndrome (IBS). As a possible therapy for irritable bowel syndrome (IBS), immune modulators such as anti-TNF-alpha drugs and anti-IL-12/23 medicines are now under investigation.

Nutritional supplements: There is preliminary evidence that some dietary supplements, including peppermint oil, psyllium, and probiotics, may be useful in the management of IBS symptoms.

Cognitive behavioral therapy: Cognitive behavioral therapy, sometimes known as CBT, is a kind of talk therapy that aims to assist patients in altering the unhelpful patterns of thinking and behaving that are holding them back. Research has demonstrated that cognitive behavioral therapy (CBT) is useful in lowering the symptoms of irritable bowel syndrome (IBS) by assisting patients in better managing their stress and anxiety.

The prognosis for those who suffer from IBS

Since IBS is a chronic illness that may be well controlled with a mix of lifestyle adjustments, medicine, and other treatments, the prognosis for persons who have been diagnosed with the condition is typically optimistic. Nevertheless, it is essential to keep in mind that irritable bowel syndrome is an extremely personalized disease, and as a result, treatments that are effective for one person may not be effective for another. Finding the most successful therapy method could need some time spent experimenting with different strategies.

It is also essential to have a clear understanding that irritable bowel syndrome (IBS) may be treated, but it may not be cured. Even with medication, irritable bowel syndrome (IBS) may cause symptoms to reappear at irregular intervals in some patients. Yet, individuals who have IBS may attain a decent quality of life and reduce the influence that their symptoms have on their lives by working closely with healthcare specialists and using effective ways of living with their condition.

There is reason to have optimism for the development of novel therapies and a deeper understanding of IBS as research on the illness continues to make progress. It is vital for individuals who have irritable bowel syndrome (IBS) to work closely with their healthcare providers to build a customized treatment plan and to make sure that they are up to speed on the most recent research and breakthroughs in the management of IBS.

CONCLUSION

Irritable Bowel Syndrome (IBS) is a condition that may make daily life difficult, but it is vital to keep in mind that there are methods to manage the condition and get relief from its symptoms.

If you have any reason to believe that you may have irritable bowel syndrome (IBS), you should make an appointment with a medical professional as soon as possible so that a diagnosis can be made and a treatment strategy may be developed that is suited to your requirements. Alterations to one's lifestyle, such as those brought about by the use of stress-reduction strategies, alterations to one's nutrition, the use of various drugs, or participation in alternative treatment modalities are all

Consuming food that is good for you and well-balanced is a key component of IBS symptom management. Working with a licensed dietitian who can give recommendations on which foods to include and which to avoid, as well as techniques for meal planning and preparation, may be useful. Dietitians may be found at the American Dietetic Association.

It is also essential to take care of your mental health, since worry and stress may make the symptoms of irritable bowel syndrome (IBS) worse. Think about implementing stress reduction practices into your daily routine, such as mindfulness, meditation, or yoga; alternatively, seek the help of a mental health professional.

Keep in mind that you do not stand alone. You may connect with people who are going through experiences similar to yours and benefit from the various resources that are available to assist you in managing your symptoms. Your healthcare physician may give advice and support throughout your journey with irritable bowel syndrome (IBS), and support groups and online forums can be an excellent opportunity to share your experiences and learn from those of other people.

It is possible to live a full and satisfying life with irritable bowel syndrome (IBS) if the appropriate therapy and self-care measures are used.

If you suffer from irritable bowel syndrome (IBS), it is essential to collaborate closely with your healthcare practitioner to identify a treatment strategy that is effective for you. Alterations to one's way of life, medicine, and complementary or alternative treatments might all be part of the solution. In addition to taking care of your physical health, it is essential to discover effective strategies to deal with mental health issues such as stress and worry.

Having irritable bowel syndrome (IBS) may be difficult to manage, but it is vital to keep in mind that you are not the only one dealing with this condition. There is a wealth of information, guidance, and emotional support that can be obtained from a variety of sites, including in-person support groups and online forums. Many individuals who have irritable bowel syndrome can control their symptoms and lead lives that are meaningful when they get the appropriate therapy and support.

The following is a summary of the most important information that is presented in this book on irritable bowel syndrome (IBS):

- Irritable bowel syndrome (IBS) is a common gastrointestinal disorder that affects the functioning of the large intestine and can cause symptoms such as abdominal pain, bloating, and changes in bowel habits. Although the exact cause of IBS is unknown, factors such as diet, stress, and abnormal gut motility are thought to contribute to its development. IBS can be classified into three main types based on the predominant symptoms: IBS with constipation (IBS-C), and IBS with diarrhea (IBS-M).

- Irritable bowel syndrome (IBS) is often diagnosed by evaluating a patient's symptoms and ruling out other illnesses that can produce similar symptoms.

- Modifications to one's diet and stress management techniques may be helpful in the treatment of irritable bowel syndrome symptoms.

- Antispasmodics and laxatives are two examples of the kind of medications that a doctor could provide to treat certain symptoms.

- Complementary therapy for irritable bowel syndrome (IBS) may include the use of alternative therapies like acupuncture and probiotics.

- The low FODMAP diet has been demonstrated to be useful in treating symptoms of irritable bowel syndrome (IBS) for some individuals, however, it is important to follow this diet under the supervision of a qualified medical professional.

- Those who suffer from irritable bowel syndrome have access to tools and support groups that may assist them in managing the symptoms of their disease.

Continuous research is being carried out to find novel therapies for irritable bowel syndrome (IBS) and get a deeper understanding of the processes that underlie the disorder.